Other products available from Stephanie Sewell
at www.StephanieSewell.com:

Fit Happens with Know Exercise! 28 Days of Success for Every Body
5 STEPS to a Healthier You Exercise DVD
5 STEPS to a Healthier You: Kids Boot Camp Edition Exercise DVD
Cardio in 5 (a four-disc audio cardiovascular workout program)

FIT HAPPENS
with NUTRITION!

Four Weeks of Success for Every Toddler

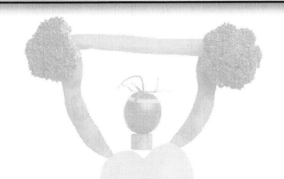

STEPHANIE HILTON SEWELL

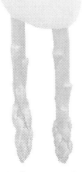

iUniverse, Inc.
Bloomington

Fit Happens with Nutrition!
Four Weeks of Success for Every Toddler

iUniverse books may be ordered through booksellers or by contacting:

iUniverse
1663 Liberty Drive
Bloomington, IN 47403
www.iuniverse.com
1-800-Authors (1-800-288-4677)

ISBN: 978-1-4620-4221-0 (sc)
ISBN: 978-1-4620-4222-7 (e)

Printed in the United States of America

iUniverse rev. date: 8/30/2011

This book is dedicated to my husband Darric Sewell, my parents Welborn and Shannon Hilton, and my extended family for always supporting me emotionally and spiritually.

I want to give a special thank you to Dariel, Belk Elizabeth, and David Hilton Sewell for showing me how to be a cool mom. I love and cherish all of you. You have been an inspiration to me, and I will continue to motivate and encourage you to be your best!

The Toddler's Affirmation

I want the world to see
That I will do what is best for me
I will play, laugh, and have fun with you
I will eat my fruit and veggies too!
By doing this, the world will see
That this is what is best for me!

—Stephanie Sewell

Contents

Introduction

After writing my first book, *Fit Happens with Know Exercise!: 28 Days of Success for Every Body*, I literally hit the road, juggling a packed schedule of fitness bootcamps and speaking engagements. After I had tackled and survived the writing process, it was such an exhilarating experience to meet people who were interested in taking on my personal plan as their own weight-management strategy.

At one engagement, I met a gentleman who wanted to ask me a question concerning his daughter. I could see that he was extremely overweight and living an unhealthy lifestyle. Even though I wanted to address his overall health and wellness goals first, I listened to his question. He began by saying, "My daughter loves to eat." I can recall the anguish on his face as he slowly and emphatically spoke the words. "I know she gets that bad habit from me, and I have to make a change for both of our sakes."

It was heartbreaking, but I realized then the important role parents play in setting healthy examples for their children to follow, whether it's treating friends and family members with respect, teaching and modeling good manners, or providing and indulging in healthy meals and nutritious snacks that are appropriate and nourishing for active lifestyles and growing bodies.

Obesity is on the rise in the United States, and I was appalled to learn that the children's sections of many department stores now carry prominently displayed plus-sized clothing. More teenagers than ever before are dealing with weight-related issues like heart disease, diabetes, and a whole host of issues that threaten to do serious, long-term damage to their self-esteem.

As the mother of a toddler, I realized that it is never too early to teach a child to eat the right foods, in a variety of textures and colors, and in the right portion sizes. When I thought of that father and his daughter, I couldn't help but wonder how different their lives could have been if they had taken a different path toward healthier lifestyles. What would happen if we *all* took more responsibility for teaching our children while they're young about healthy eating habits?

My daughter watches everything I do, and every child is influenced by every observation. I'm teaching her how to indulge in nutritious, colorful foods, and showing her good examples that I hope will inform her eating decisions for the rest of her life. I have to share those lessons with you, and *every* parent, who is truly committed to giving his or her child the very best life he or she can live. Thank you for using *Fit Happens with Nutrition* with your toddler!

The Reason Behind My Madness!

Attention all Parents: this is your official wake-up call! Beyond that, this is a *call to action* on behalf of your little loved one. Countless studies have confirmed that a child's first five years of life are a critical mental and physical development period. The habits they are exposed to in these early years can, and will, set the stage for the rest of their lives. Before continuing, we have to discuss a few musts for every parent who reads *Fit Happens with Nutrition!: Four Weeks of Success for Every Toddler*.

I can't say it enough: parents must take responsibility for every bite of food their children eat. It's just that simple! The school your child attends is not at fault, especially if your child is eating only one meal there—lunch—and breakfast and dinner are provided at home.

Parents must be parents *all the time*. What does that mean? It means not giving in to the drive-thru solution on a daily basis. We're all living fast-paced, eat-on-the-go lives, and it can be so easy to just pull into the drive-thru lane of your favorite fast-food restaurant. This book can show you some easy ways to plan meals at home and prepare take-along snacks that allow for valuable learning moments with your child … and help you save the drive-thru for special treats!

Parents must be aware of the healthy tools at their disposal to help their children learn the basics of good nutrition. This book features the tools you'll need to start your child on the right path of learning healthy habits and recognizing healthy options away from home. The transition from baby foods to table foods is a big step, so let's take it together!

In *Fit Happens with Know Exercise*, I explained how to establish healthy new habits that lead to positive and lasting lifestyle changes. What I will share in this book will help you to create and reinforce healthy habits for your own child, and you can rest assured that everything here comes directly from my home to yours. No two children are exactly alike, but every child enjoys learning. For children between the ages of eighteen months and five years, every day is an adventure, and parents must be fully engaged!

I'm so glad you have chosen to take on this adventure in healthy eating! Let's begin the journey together!

Learn Your ABCs: A Bullying Chapter

It's hard to believe that your sweet little boy or girl is very likely to be one of three things: a witness to bullying, a participant in or instigator of bullying, or the victim of bullying. It might be even more amazing to realize that your child could actually be learning the basics of bullying—how to use and react to hurtful words or intimidating situations—directly from *you.*

While bullies can't claim a certain magical age when they come into being, they certainly get an early start in their overall development by absorbing cues at a young age. Young children are highly impressionable and tune in closely to emotional situations. They absorb the energy and commotion of a car chase on television; they observe the interactions between their peers when it's time to share a toy; and they listen to how their family members relate to each other during a disagreement. Your children are watching *every* action and *every* reaction.

If Daddy laughs at something funny, the child will make an immediate connection: "Daddy thinks that is funny, so that is funny to me, too." Or, if Mommy describes an object a certain way, the child will think, "Mommy said it, so it must be true."

Now consider how a child is affected when Daddy finds it funny to point out and joke about people who are overweight or when Mommy says the neighbor is nice but should "lay off the sweets." Young children hear those words, internalize them, and sooner rather than later, the words grow into ugly, hurtful remarks they will repeat.

Remember, our children are gardens, and we, parents, are farmers. Every lesson we teach, every meal we serve, every action (and reaction) we show our children, and every word we speak into their lives is like fertilizer that we add to our little gardens. Are you cultivating a child who can see the beauty, diversity, and value of every person? Or, is your child growing into someone intolerant, selfish, and insensitive to others' feelings?

Your child is the ultimate reflection of the effort you sow into his or her life. Now is the time to put good stuff in by watching your words, paying attention to your own actions, and helping your child to resolve conflicts and intimidating situations with confidence and thoughtful solutions. Sticks and stones *can* break big and little bones, and words *can* hurt feelings, self-esteem, and so much more.

WEEK 1:
Colors of the Rainbow

Welcome to Week 1! Colors are all around your little one, and each day brings those colors into clearer focus. That's lemon yellow, mud-pie brown, and every color in between. Each day of this week will be devoted to a specific color and examples you will easily find around the house, in your own pantry, or along one of the aisles in your favorite grocery store.

Day 1:
Make This a Red-Color Day!

Let's kick things off with a little excitement! Introducing your little one to healthy, nutritious food is an important milestone you can achieve on a daily basis. Today, we'll set the tone with the color red and encourage eating a few delicious fruits and vegetables: juicy strawberries and red grapes, crisp red onions, sweet red beets and pomegranates, garden-fresh tomatoes, red-skin potatoes, and mouth-watering watermelon.

These wonderful reds are packed with antioxidants, the "security guards" that keep our cells from getting damaged by disease-causing bacteria. In today's delicious red harvest, the antioxidants can help the body fight off several forms of cancer and heart disease.

Begin by showing your child the actual fruit or vegetable. Hold it in your hand, and then let your child hold it. Allow your child to explore its size and shape. This will hold your child's attention while you work at the kitchen counter to slice a piece for tasting.

Next, place the whole fruit or vegetable next to the sliced pieces and begin your tasting time. Use descriptions while you share the experience with your child: *Look at the juicy red strawberry! The slices look like little red hearts. Don't they taste sweet?*

It's very important that your child sees you enjoying the tasting experience. Children are natural mimics, and during the toddler and preschool years, they imitate the actions of their siblings, their peers, and the adults who are closest to them. For fruits and vegetables you haven't tasted before or you feel a little unsure about trying, this is a great time to try something new and share a wonderful experience with your child.

HEALTHY TIP: Reinforce the tasting time by taking a trip to the library and finding books about fruits and vegetables, or books that feature fruits and vegetables as characters.

Day 2:
Let's Sing the Blues, Baby!

A ny chance to share a positive experience with your child is something worth singing about, so let's sing the blues ... more like the blues and the purples, to be exact!

Introduce your child to a handful of fresh blueberries, ripe purple plums, delicious raspberries and blackberries, purple grapes and raisins, eggplant, and figs (the real thing). Studies have shown that these dark blue and purple fruits and vegetables also contain antioxidants. As we discussed on Red-Color Day, the little security guards in these fruits and vegetables also protect our cells from damage, help the brain's memory center to stay healthy, and protect against cancer and heart disease.

For today's tasting time, most of these fruits are great for little hands to hold. They also make excellent counting tools! Describe the fruit and encourage your child to sample it at the same time: *Let's eat these three yummy little blueberries! One yummy blueberry, two yummy blueberries, and three yummy blueberries are all gone. Time for some more!*

Don't forget to show your child how much you are enjoying this experience. Those little eyes are watching your every move, so keep the nutritious beat moving and sing the blues loud and clear!

HEALTHY TIP: Reinforce today's tasting time by selecting a blue or purple fruit or vegetable and using it in a snack recipe, as a mealtime side item, or in a dessert.

Day 3:
Let's Go Green!

Green is more than a buzzword—it's a way of life, and it's one of the best ways to eat! Gorgeous green fruits and vegetables are easy to spot and just as easy to include in meals and snacks. Green apples, green grapes, broccoli, and cool honeydew melon are all delicious and ready to eat right after being washed. Green beans and leafy greens, such as kale, spinach, and turnip, mustard, and collard greens, add texture and flavor to any meal.

Many green fruits and vegetables contain lutein, which helps promote eye health, and folate, a B vitamin that helps to prevent birth defects. Moms-to-be shouldn't miss out on any of this green goodness!

Today's tasting time can include three bowls of any green fruit or vegetable you'd like to introduce your child to: *First, we'll taste the sliced green grapes. Now, let's taste the crunchy green bell pepper slices. And this bowl of sweet green apple slices? We can dip them in the yummy yogurt!*

HEALTHY TIP: Reinforce today's tasting time by visiting the grocery store or a farmer's market and letting your child pick out all of the green fruits and vegetables.

Day 4:
Life's an Orange ... It's So A-Peeling!

Every day, your toddler is learning so much about the world and absorbing it all in the most amazing way. Young children love to see, hear, touch, taste, and smell their way around. The whole world might as well be orange—it's all so a-peeling!

Among orange fruits and vegetables, oranges top the list and are joined by cantaloupes, papayas, carrots, butternut squash, sweet potatoes, and pumpkins. Citrus fruits like oranges, tangerines, and mandarins are great sources of vitamin C, which helps little bodies (and big ones, too!) maintain strong immune systems. Yams, sweet potatoes, pumpkins, and carrots contain beta-carotene, which the body converts to vitamin A. Vitamin A promotes eye health and strong mucous membranes. It also plays a role in keeping cancer, heart disease, and high cholesterol at bay. Sound familiar?

Take a different turn with this tasting time and explore the skins of each orange fruit or vegetable: *The juicy orange has a peel that protects the fruit inside. See how you can pull the slices apart? The sweet potato has a thin skin that gets flaky when we bake it in the oven. See how it looks mushy and orange inside?*

HEALTHY TIP: Reinforce today's tasting time by lining up an orange, a sweet potato, a carrot, and a pumpkin and then testing how they roll down a ramp made from your cutting board.

5

Day 5:
Hello, Yellow!

Like sunshine on a summer day, yellow fruits and vegetables make the body smile all over! They are the brightest picks for the dinner plate and pack a can't-miss dose of nutrients for growing bodies.

Lemons, yellow peppers, bananas, peaches, mangoes, yellow squash, zucchini, and sweet corn are all fruits and vegetables that don't require a lot of preparation before they become delicious snacks or mealtime sides. Similar to the a-peeling orange group, these yellow selections also pack in vitamins A and C for a one-two punch against eye diseases, heart disease, and reducing the risk of birth defects.

Ditch the mellow approach to yellow tasting time and add a blindfold: *Show me the yellow lemon and then show me the yellow corn. Now that I can't see, feed me the yellow lemon. Wow! That yellow lemon is so sour!*

HEALTHY TIP: Reinforce today's tasting time by comparing the yellow corn to the yellow squash, or a yellow lemon to a mango.

Day 6:
Bringing It All Together

A healthy meal includes at least three different colors of foods on the plate. This week, you've shared a whole rainbow of nutritious choices with your child; and hopefully, you've also expanded your own ideas toward incorporating more of these delicious options into every meal and snack.

Parent and child assignment: Find three colors from this week and put them all together for one meal.
Example 1: Create a fruit salad including mandarin orange slices, juicy red strawberries, and a few fresh blueberries.
Example 2: Make sure dinner includes a leafy green spinach salad, an entrée of orange or lemon chicken, and a side of red-skin potatoes.

Items Needed

_____

_____

_____

_____

_____

Day 7:
Sharing Is Caring
Share what you have learned with your family and friends.

I t's time for you and your child to celebrate! You've made it through a whole week of rainbow eating! The lessons you've learned and shared by tasting a variety of fruits and vegetables will be the foundation for a lifetime of healthy choices. Take the next step with the fruits and vegetables you and your child have tasted this week and use them in other recipes or combine them in creative snacks. You get extra credit for a smoothie that includes juicy red strawberries, delicious yellow pineapple chunks, and a splash of orange juice!

Today, take the opportunity to share this week's lessons with a loved one. Help your child to look through newspapers or magazines to find their favorite fruits and vegetables from this week. Use what you both find to create a collage of your favorite fruits and vegetables and help them explain it to aunts, a cousin, a grandparent, or a family friend.

Then let your child select their favorite fruit or vegetable in the collage as a snack time treat. Don't be surprised if they can't choose just one—that just means you've done an *excellent* job!

Activity for Today

_____

_____

_____

_____

_____

WEEK 2:
What Is Your Shape?

Welcome to Week 2! I would like to thank you and your little one for taking the next great big step on our nutritious journey! This week is shaping up to be loaded with variety: a special treat for little minds that are always thinking!

Just for a moment, I'd like you to sit down on the floor and look around the room. Did the whole world suddenly get a whole lot bigger? That's your child's current view of the world. It's easy to forget that when you're holding small fingers or picking up your little sweetie for a squirmy hug. All week long, we're going to work on easy ways to help your little one embrace a variety of shapes. We're going to focus on the big, the little, the round, the square, and the yummy zig-zags and odd shapes of healthy eating!

Day 8:
Round

Aside from colors, shapes are among the first lessons we teach our children. Why not take the lesson into the kitchen and right onto their plates?

Use any mealtime (breakfast, lunch, or dinner) to point out the shapes that are being prepared. When you open the can of "round green peas," let your little one help you pour them into the pan. On your cutting board, show your child the sliced carrots that are "orange circles." For a double dose of round, cut a circular hole in an orange, and then plug the hole. Show your child the "round orange," let her remove the "little circle." Then help her squeeze out the juice for a sip from her "round orange cup."

TODDLER TIP: One of the easiest round shapes our little ones recognize is a Cheerio. This cereal is an excellent source of whole grains and the perfect size for little fingers that are just learning to pick things up without assistance. A good way to reinforce their shape is to hold one between your thumb and index finger and then show your child how to roll the Cheerio like a wheel. Add a little "vroom-vroom" sound effect and pop it in your mouth! You can easily create a game with your child or just hold their attention with your sound effects.

Day 9:
Square

Today, it's so hip to be square! Did you know that the origin of the term "square meal" dates back to the 1600s? Over time, it has come to refer to a healthy, balanced meal—exactly what you want for your child!

Square menu ideas aren't hard to find, especially when we begin with breakfast. Try a square waffle and help your little one count the squares! Remember not to drown the waffle with calorie-laden syrup. Play a game of four-square and let your child pick any four squares to fill with syrup. If you're serving toast, try cutting the big square into four little squares, making it a little easier for little fingers to handle.

Dare to be square!

TODDLER TIP: At lunch or snack time, serve cheese cubes with a light ranch dip, a few carrot and celery sticks, and tasty wheat or graham crackers. At dinner, consider cutting your child's meat into orderly squares and then getting them to count each bite. It's never too early to work in a little counting practice!

Day 10:
Big and Little

It's a BIG deal to focus on the little details of healthy eating! Children learn and absorb more information about their world between birth and five years of age than at any other point in their lives. An important part of their learning begins when they start comparing shapes and sizes, especially opposites like big and little.

When you're out and about, take every opportunity to point out the differences in sizes. At the grocery store, compare the big head of lettuce to the little artichoke. If you eat lunch in a restaurant, talk about your own big glass of water and your child's small cup of water.

TODDLER TIP: At mealtime or snack time, show the difference between eating a big bite and a little bite, then let your child point out some big and little examples on their own plate. You'll be amazed by the big impact of so many little lessons!

Day 11:
Little and Big

Yes, we're revisiting little and big, but this time we're adding a twist: let's talk about little and big portion sizes!

It's no secret that the amount of food we consume in the United States has definitely grown over the past twenty years. The staggering rates of obesity across all age groups are evidence of this fact. The average restaurant entrée is served in an amount that can adequately feed two diners or fill one diner, with enough left over to take home. (Check out the appendix for more information about Nutrition Facts labeling and understanding serving sizes.)

I want you to try this: look at your open hand, make a fist, and then hold it. Your fist is about the size of your own stomach. The same goes for your own child's little fist. Their fist is about the same size as their stomach. Now think of what has to happen to get a big amount of food into such a little space! Now is the perfect time to pay attention to portion sizes and serving sizes whenever you read food labels.

TODDLER TIP: At today's snack time, set out a correct serving size of potato chips and a large serving. Talk about how the little serving is just right to fill up a little tummy, and how a big serving looks yummy, but will get a little tummy too full and make it hurt. Be sure to explain that the same thing can happen to grown-up tummies, too.

Day 12:
Odd Shapes

Just what is an odd-shaped food? To your child, that could be any dish that doesn't fit any of the standard shapes but is still a nutritious option that shouldn't be missed. Every parent who takes on Day 12 has to be committed to making this a fun day of learning *and* possibly conquering some foods he or she has personally avoided.

Children look up to their parents and watch closely for their reactions to every situation. When your little one stubs their toe, they will run to you for comfort, but they also are looking for your reaction. If you're calm and soothing about the pain of that toe, they will know everything will be alright. The same goes for that plate of squiggly spaghetti and tomato sauce, good sources of grains and lycopenes, respectively. If you take a bite of a new food and explain how good it is, your child will be more likely to at least give the dish a try. Here are some tips on tackling oddly shaped vegetables:

Asparagus: This spear-shaped vegetable (which also looks like a little tree) is a good source of iron, magnesium, and zinc. It works well when served with a dip, rather than alone or sliced.

Beets: The root and leaves are both delicious additions to any meal. The red root, rich in fiber and folates, can be boiled and sliced into rounds, then cut into half-moons or "smiles" for your little one to gobble up.

Brussels Sprouts: This vegetable features protein content in addition to being a source of vitamins A and C. Though this vegetable may appear bite-sized to an adult, keep in mind that a little mouth may be overstuffed by the attempt! For best results, steam these sprouts, then slice two or three for easy chewing.

TODDLER TIP: Avoid scary food descriptions and stick with focusing on how the dish tastes and how it will help your child grow big and strong. Also, keep your child's plate simple at mealtime. If an entrée features a thick gravy or sauce, try placing a small amount in a side dish or bowl and allow your child to dip his or her meat or vegetables, rather than watch them refuse to eat anything at all.

Day 13:
Bringing It All Together

We've covered quite a bit of ground, and I'm proud of you for sticking with it! I hope you noticed that your child was more observant about the food you were eating this week and that you were able to share some new food experiences.

As you engage your child with new foods or even some old favorites, be sure to work in positive comparisons that help make connections.

Examples:
These sliced carrots look like the wheels of Mommy's car!
These pasta shells look just like the seashells Daddy found at the beach.

Here's an idea you can use to really tie things together: play the "human shape-up" game! Challenge your child to do their best imitation of a shape using yoga stretches. You'll both get a calorie-burning workout while having a little fun!

Example:
When you say, "Make yourself into a round Cheerio," your child will assume the shape of a circle.
When you say, "Shape your body into a cheese cube," your child will assume the shape of a box.
(See appendix II for examples of body poses as a resource.)

What shapes did you make?

_____

_____

_____

_____

_____

15

Day 14:
Sharing and Caring

H ooray! You and your child have officially conquered a week full of food shapes! This week's lessons actually did double duty: They helped to strengthen your little's one recognition of common shapes. They also reinforced the unspoken lesson that differences are everywhere, and they really do taste good! Ultimately, I want you and your child to be open to the delicious differences that add necessary variety to any diet.

Today, take the opportunity to let your child show what he or she has learned. Go through your pantry, kitchen cupboards, and refrigerator shelves together and look for different food shapes. Your child will be amazed to see uncooked spaghetti, hear the shake of dry oats that are usually creamy mush, or see leafy green kale before it is steamed.

Let your child pick one or two nonperishable items that can be donated to a local food bank or soup kitchen and then follow up to actually drop off the items. Explain to your child that everyone deserves to eat healthy, nutritious food, in all shapes and sizes, and that sharing what we have with others gives us a great big heart!

Items Needed

_____

_____

_____

_____

_____

WEEK 3:
Texture and Taste

Welcome to Week 3. Go ahead and pat yourself on the back! This week, I want you to introduce your little one to food texture and taste. Texture is the feeling of the food in your mouth, right after you taste it but before you chew it and swallow. For your little one, feeling food texture is a brand-new experience, especially as he or she is still learning to negotiate solid foods.

Taste is pretty simple—it's the sensation of flavor as defined by your tongue's taste buds, which number in the thousands! Specific regions of the tongue contain groups of taste buds that are more sensitive to sweet, sour, bitter, or salty tastes. Exposure to cultural influences and seasoning preferences help determine what tastes and textures will ultimately appeal to young eaters.

Texture and taste also represent another opportunity for parents to make peace with foods that occupy an unpleasant place in a childhood memory or experience. Remember, your own child is a clean slate. Your food prejudices can become his or her prejudices, and you owe your child the chance to really taste a food item and create his or her own experience.

So, what are we waiting for? Let's get on with the weeklong tasting party!

Day 15:
Crunchy

Crunchy foods are action foods! They engage the jaw muscles, they rev up the saliva glands, and they set digestion in motion. The sensation of crunching is one of the most satisfying elements of eating, and getting early experience with the right types of crunchy foods can set your child on the right path to a lifetime of healthy eating.

What are the right types of crunchy foods? Raw fruits and vegetables are the best examples: delicious apples, fresh slices of bell pepper, carrots, and celery sticks provide a nutritious crunch any time. Since toddlers love to snack, also consider whole-grain crackers, pretzel sticks, and baked pita chips as options.

A word of advice: Just say no to popcorn at this stage! It's a healthy snack for older children and grown-ups but still a bit complex for toddlers. It's also too easy to get stuck on the wrong track with buttery, high-calorie versions.

ACTIVITY TIME: When serving crunchy side items or snacks, share the wisdom of chewing food thoroughly with your little one. It's a great time to start teaching the importance of proper, comprehensive chewing to aid digestion and to help your child enjoy eating.

Example:
Chant this rhyme to the tune of "Row, Row, Row Your Boat at least three times: "Take one bite, then chew-chew-chew it up; chew it really well! Chew and chew and chew and chew until I feel so swell!"

While your child will think, *Yea!! A chewing game and a song to sing!*, you'll actually be setting the stage for enjoying crunchy snacks at a leisurely pace!

Day 16:
Mushy

Mmmm, mmmm, mushy! Doesn't it seem like just yesterday when mushy foods were the only ones that your little one knew? But mushy foods aren't all reserved for the baby food stage.

What comes to mind when you think of mushy foods? How about delicious applesauce, sliced bananas, oatmeal with cinnamon, creamy twice-baked potatoes, a smooth bowl of yogurt, or cool fruit smoothies? There are plenty of healthy options—and even more when you apply your creativity to your blender!

Because mushy foods are soft, they don't take as much work as crunchy foods to chew. When introducing these foods, its still a good idea to be cautious and teach good chewing habits that lead to smooth digestion.

ACTIVITY TIME: Help your little one to resist taking a few good chews and then swallowing everything semi-whole. Show your child how to take a small bite and hum our chewing song: "Take one bite, then chew-chew-chew it up; chew it really well! Chew and chew and chew and chew until I feel so swell!" (Hum the tune of "Row, Row, Row Your Boat at least two times.)

Consider pairing a mushy food item and another food with a solid texture, like yogurt and apple slices. Allow your little one to experience each texture separately and then together.

Day 17:
Sweet

W hat could be sweeter than being with your little one? Teaching him or her to have the right attitude toward sweet foods and sweets in general!

Sweet tastes are some of the first tastes we encounter—and then it's love at first mouthful! While desserts, candy, and artificially sweetened drinks are obvious sweets, parents should also keep an eye on fruit juice with 100 percent juice content, the extra addition of refined (white) sugar to recipes, and the sugar content in many snacks.

Use moderation with sweets and any food item you introduce to your child. It's quite alright to let your child see you enjoy something sweet from time to time. Remember, your child is watching your reaction to everything. If you are interested in eating a lot of sweets, your child will be, too!

ACTIVITY TIME: When introducing sweets to your child, take a balanced approach. Most fruits, like juicy strawberries, mango chunks, peaches, nectarines, and watermelon feature natural sugars, which growing bodies need for fuel. Add a serving or two with each meal, or serve as a snack during the day. Cupcakes and cookies are fine; just keep them in mind as special treats and not a part of your toddler's daily diet. If you are trying to control your own sweet tooth, consider using applesauce or honey as a guilt-free replacement sweetener in cupcake, quick bread, and cookie recipes.

Day 18:
Salty

Salty tastes are unmistakable! Most foods don't start out being salty; salt is added as a flavoring.

In the case of some meats, like ham, bacon, or beef or turkey jerky, the salt (or sodium chloride, for you label readers) is used as a preservative. It's a good idea to watch the amount of sodium chloride you encounter in your child's snacks and in foods prepared for the family. Taking in too much salt has a direct impact on heart and kidney health across all age groups.

ACTIVITY TIME: What's the best way to introduce salt to your little one? Allow him or her to taste a bit from the saltshaker and to see the salt crystals themselves on a plate or napkin. Explain that salt is added to soup or to bitter foods (more on those tomorrow!) to help them taste better.

Day 19:
Bitter

J ust the thought of a bitter food item is enough to make me squeeze my eyes shut and shudder! We'll set those thoughts aside and forge ahead to this challenging yet essential taste!

Bitter foods include quince, cranberries, and grapefruit. It is tempting to lump in sour foods, such as lemons, with the bitter foods; however, the tastes are a little different. Both sour and bitter foods are complemented by salty or sweet flavorings to improve overall taste.

ACTIVITY TIME: When you introduce a bitter food item, prepare one small portion in its natural state and then prepare another portion with a flavoring. Serve the natural portion first and get your child to share how he or she feels about the food and its taste. Then serve the next portion and explain it as a different way to eat the same food. Again, encourage your child to share how he or she feels about the food and its taste. Work hard to keep your own reactions evenly balanced so your little one forms an opinion of his or her own.

Day 20:
Bringing It All Together

W hat a week! I'm proud of you for hanging in there! By exploring textures and different tastes, we've ventured into the next dimension of eating. These are the nuances that normally go unspoken and are passed along by a parent's preference or a cultural or religious influence. By expanding your child's experience with texture and tastes, you have widened their eating experience and given him or her vocabulary to complement this week's lessons!

Consider preparing a "blind feast" to test what your little one has learned! Prepare a serving in each of the categories covered this week: crunchy, mushy, sweet, salty, and bitter. Have your child cover his or her eyes while sampling a serving and attempting to identify the food and describe how it tastes. Alternate with your child by tasting one of the servings yourself!

Items Needed

_____

_____

_____

_____

_____

Day 21:
Sharing and Caring

I t's hard to believe that we've reached this part of our journey! You and your child have experienced a treasure trove of nutritious eating, and you should really celebrate this milestone!

Today, consider sharing this week's experiences with someone who serves in the military. One of the many things soldiers miss when they are stationed abroad includes the tastes and textures of foods. Help your child select three of this week's tastes and textures and create a gift basket.

Example:
At the grocery store or in your own pantry, your child selects pretzels, beef jerky, and cookies. Allow your child to make a greeting card or a thank-you card for the soldier and present the gift to the local USO, recruiting office, or Armed Forces support center.

Items Needed

_____

_____

_____

_____

_____

WEEK 4:
Food Groups

Welcome to Week 4—give yourself a hand! You and your little one have covered a lot of concepts, and now it's time to blend them all together like a cool, refreshing smoothie!

Until recently, I'm sure that when you heard someone say "food groups," you thought of the "four food groups" and the basic elements of good nutrition. The US Department of Agriculture (USDA) changed the way nutrition is explained by introducing the Food Guide Pyramid in 2005 in order to do a better job of sharing information with Americans about how to make healthy, nutritious choices. In June 2011, a new model was introduced, called MyPlate (see chart).

What used to be known as the milk/dairy group, the meat group, the breads/grains group, and the fruits/vegetables group has changed in order to reflect more balanced meals in healthy, appropriate portion sizes. MyPlate features fruits and vegetables in separate groups, gathers meat, beans, fish, and nuts together into the protein group, and places bread, breakfast cereals, pasta, oatmeal, rice, and tortillas into the grains group.

Overall, MyPlate provides a clear path to healthy food choices and serves up a generous portion of visual appeal for grown-ups and children as you follow the steps to creating a colorful, nutritious meal at every meal time. Now, are you and your little one ready to sample a helping of MyPlate's portions? Ready, set, GO ... to a great week of learning about MyPlate!

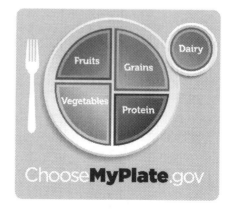

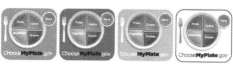

Day 22:
Protein

O ur main sources of protein include beef, pork, poultry (chicken and turkey), fish, and eggs. While we can spend a lot of time discussing topic, I really want you to understand that all of these sources have something in common: they can all serve as a key serving of protein in a balanced diet.

Within MyPlate, proteins include beans, which are another excellent source of protein. We'll talk more about beans on Day 23. When you are preparing a meat selection for an entrée or as one part of your family's overall meal, focus on selecting meats that are lean and low-fat.

While we've all had the "get something quick from the drive-thru" experience, pay close attention to those bits of chicken your little one loves so much. Chicken gets the spotlight, because it is most likely sold in a quick-serve format. Fish sticks have the chance to shine for the same reason. Limit your child's intake of breaded meats and look for choices that are grilled, baked, or broiled.

Picky eater advice: you may need to get your little one to experiment with meat options. Through many trials and a few errors, my own daughter was introduced to each type of meat. Now we know that as long as chicken hot dog franks, baked chicken, and grilled fish are around, we can't go wrong!

TASTING PARTY: As I mentioned earlier, try not to bring any of your own "food baggage" into the experimenting.* Allow your little one to taste every type of meat and gain a better understanding of the differences. Try cutting up two or three types of meat, such as a serving of diced chicken, a few sliced rounds of a hotdog (beef or turkey frank), or few tender flakes of a fish fillet (boneless is best). Place them on separate plates and let your little one taste each meat. Taste each piece along with your child and note his or her reaction.

*I understand that religious or dietary restrictions may take priority at mealtime. I don't endorse one meat source above another. I do encourage every parent to make wise and healthy decisions and seek information about nutrition content for any food being introduced to children.

Day 23:
Beans

Beans! Beans! They're good for your heart ... and they keep some other important bodily functions in good working condition! As I indicated on Day 22, beans and peas make up a significant segment of MyPlate. We can list a wide variety of beans, but I primarily want you to remember that beans include dry beans or peas, nuts, and seeds.*

Just what are dry beans? These are legumes that include black beans, lima beans, black-eyed peas, chickpeas, lentils, pinto beans, and kidney beans, to name a few. As vegetables with natural plant proteins, beans also come packed with zinc and iron, which are important for growing strong bones and muscles. Beans are highly nutritious and can, in some cases, count as a substitute for meat sources.

Don't think that you have to serve your little one a plate of plain old beans. Get creative! Consider serving black bean soup, hummus (made from chickpeas and tahini, a sesame seed paste), or chili with or without the meat source of your choice and spice up the menu!

TASTING PARTY: Just about any bean is perfect finger food for your little one! Try serving a few red kidney beans, a few cut green beans, and a few black-eyed peas. Start by cutting one or two of each in half, so you and your child can see how they look on the inside. Sample each bean with your child and explain that beans can be round, long, big, or small, and can come in many different colors.

*It may be necessary to take caution with introducing your little one to nuts, as they can represent an allergen source.

Day 24:
Grains

The grains group includes any food made from oats, wheat, barley, cornmeal, rice, or another cereal grain. While the word "cereal" itself will sound as familiar as that favorite box of fun currently sitting in your pantry, breads, tortillas, grits, oatmeal, and pasta, are examples of grain products.

It's important to know that grains come in two forms: whole and refined. It's easy to remember that whole grains, like whole wheat bread and brown rice, include a whole group of nutrients: fiber, iron, and many of the B vitamins. Refined grains, like those found in white bread and white rice, have to be enriched because the nutrients are removed in the refining process. Get an early start with your little one and get him/her used to eating whole grains whenever possible.*

TASTING PARTY: Compare and contrast a whole-wheat food item with a refined-wheat item! Cook a serving of brown rice and a serving of white rice and then add a vegetable like green beans or broccoli. Show your child each dish and go over all the ways they are similar (same name, same size, etc.) and all the ways they are different (color, taste, etc.). Taste a spoonful of each along with your child and note his or her reaction.

*As with any food item, it is important for parents to make wise and healthy decisions for their children. Some grain products may present issues with digestion due to their gluten content.

Day 25:
Vegetables

The vegetable group should be very familiar. If not, just turn back to Weeks 1 and 2. Just like the produce stands at the farmer's market or the produce section of your favorite grocery store, there's a lot of variety in this group! Greens (mustard, collard, turnip, etc.), broccoli, kale, Brussels sprouts, cucumbers, carrots, okra, beans, peas, and potatoes are all delicious examples of vegetables.

Although vegetables are healthiest in their fresh, raw form, they can also be steamed, heated from a can, or bought frozen or dried/dehydrated, and served whole, cut up, or mashed.

Depending on the vegetable you serve, you'll be adding a great alphabet soup of vitamins to your little one's diet: vitamins A, B, C, E, K, and lutein, to name a few. Look for vegetables that are in season for the best mealtime options, or seek the frozen versions for year-round goodness.

TASTING PARTY: Try another compare-and-contrast activity, but this time, show your child the difference between a crunchy, raw vegetable and a soft, steamed vegetable.

Take a few sprigs of fresh broccoli and pair them with a little ranch dip; steam another serving for two or three minutes. Serve both plates to your child and explain how they are the same (broccoli, green, etc.) and how they are different (crunchy, soft, etc.) Sample a piece of each with your child and share how both versions are delicious and healthy anytime!

Day 26:
Fruits

Ahhh … the fruits group! This has to be one of my personal favorites! As a completely nutritious food you and your little one can eat *and* drink, fruit is hard to beat. This group includes apples, oranges, peaches, pears, plums, nectarines, bananas, pomegranates, blueberries, grapes, and even tomatoes! Yes, tomatoes are considered a fruit—I had to look it up myself!

Like vegetables, fruits are best when they are fresh and natural. Remember to wash all fruits thoroughly with warm water if you intend to keep the skins on when you serve them, rather than peeling the skins off. Other options include canned, frozen, or dried fruits, and they also may be served whole, cut up, or puréed.

As natural sources of vitamins A and C, fruits are some of the easiest foods to incorporate into a balanced diet. Think beyond snack time and serve sliced fruit at dinner or as an on-the-go breakfast treat when added to low-fat yogurt.

TASTING PARTY: Take two or three fruits (a kiwi, an apple, and a star fruit, for example) and slice a few pieces from the whole fruit. Set each fruit on a plate next to its slices. Show your child the original piece of fruit and then show him or her the slices and the inside of the fruit. Sample a piece of each fruit with your child and talk about which fruits are chewy, crunchy, or mushy.

Day 27:
Bringing It All Together

Wow—what a week! We've come quite a long way, and I appreciate you and your little one for being so willing to learn! This week was all about the portions represented on MyPlate, but we're not finished yet!

The dairy group includes milk, yogurt, cheese, and milk-based desserts like ice cream and puddings, and is a great source of calcium. Look for low-fat and fat-free options, as the calories in these foods can soar!

The oils group includes various cooking oils like sunflower oil, corn oil, canola oil, and olive oil. Nuts, seeds, avocados, and cooking oils contain the "good" fats. Stick margarine, shortening, lard, and butter should be limited, as these represent examples of solid or "bad" fats.

Good nutrition doesn't come easy. Healthy choices are daily choices, and I encourage you to stay open to learning about healthy options for your little one and your entire family. Take the time to get familiar with MyPlate and the foods represented in every portion. That's the best way to focus on creating the colorful plate of your own whenever you prepare a meal for your family or for yourself!

Notes

_____

_____

_____

_____

_____

Day 28:
Sharing and Caring

Trying to digest everything we've covered about MyPlate in one week is a tall order! One way to share what we've learned so that your little one will care is with an easy game you can create at home!

What you'll need:
- Six paper plates
- Two pairs of scissors (one pair for an adult, and one child's pair)
- A few magazines with lots of food pictures or a local grocery store sales paper
- A pen or a pencil

Look through the magazines and local grocery store sales paper with your little one and cut out food items that can be eaten at any meal or during any time of the day. Label the outside rim of your plates with "breakfast," "lunch," and "dinner." Arrange the food pictures you find on each plate in order to create three healthy meals based on what you've learned about MyPlate this week.

Example: Your little one creates a breakfast meal of fruit, yogurt, and a piece of toast, and you create a breakfast meal of cereal, fruit, and a piece of turkey sausage. You are helping your child recognize that there are different options that work for the same meal, and make connections about food items and the food groups they represent within MyPlate.

This fun activity will help your little one better understand the food groups, and examples of food items. Talk about sharing and caring at its best, and even parents will learn a thing or two!

Additional resources and activities from MyPlate.gov are included (See appendix III)

Notes

_____

_____

_____

About the Author

STEPHANIE SEWELL, certified personal trainer, certified group fitness instructor, certified nutrition and wellness consultant, and mom, guides her readers through *Fit Happens with Nutrition! Four Weeks of Success for Every Toddler.* Whether her readers are absolute beginners to parenting or seasoned veterans, Stephanie inspires and motivates all parents to lead by example using this daily approach to teaching the basics of good nutrition.

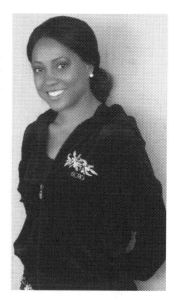

Stephanie's background includes being an inaugural member of the NFL's Carolina Panthers cheerleading squad, a former pageant titleholder (including swimsuit winner), and national fitness/figure and bikini competitor. Her most recent and proudest accomplishment is being a mom!

Stephanie knows firsthand the importance of starting early to share lessons about nutrition and believes it is the foundation for a lifetime of healthy choices. Stephanie has designed this book to share with you the secrets of nutrition success she learned as a mom.

Visit StephanieSewell.com for these additional resources:

5 STEPS to a Healthier You
5 STEPS to a Healthier You: Kids Boot Camp Edition
Cardio in 5 (a four-disc audio cardiovascular workout program)
Fit Happens with Know Exercise! 28 Days of Success for Every Body

Degree and Certifications

Stephanie obtained her BS degree from Western Carolina University. She is certified through American Fitness Professionals and Associates as an AFPA-certified personal trainer, AFPA-certified group fitness instructor, and an AFPA-certified nutrition and wellness consultant. She also works as a pharmaceutical representative specializing in diabetes care. She is a member of Toastmasters International.

The President's Council on Fitness, Sports & Nutrition (PCFSN) has chosen Stephanie Hilton Sewell to receive a 2010 PCFSN Community Leadership Award. The award is given annually to individuals who improve the lives of individuals within their community by providing or enhancing opportunities to engage in sports, physical activities, fitness or nutrition-related programs.

Competitive Accomplishments

- Miss Cherokee County (South Carolina) 1994
- Miss South Carolina America Swimsuit Preliminary Winner 1994
- Miss Spartanburg (South Carolina) USA 1997
- Miss South Carolina USA Third Runner-Up 1997
- Miss Fitness America–ESPN Top 20 Finalist 1998
- NFL Carolina Panthers Cheerleader (1996) Co-Captain
- NFL Carolina Panthers Cheerleader (1997) Captain
- NFL Carolina Panthers Cheerleader (1998) TopCat of the Year
- NFL Carolina Panthers Cheerleader (1998) ProBowl Cheerleader
- National Bikini Competition Top 10 Finalist Classic Bikini and Model America 2006
- National Bikini and Figure Competition Top 10 Finalist Classic
- Bikini and Figure Universe 2009 (Sixth and Seventh Place)
- National Physique Committee North America National Competition Masters Bikini and Open Bikini Fourth Place
- National Physique Committee Junior USA's National Competition Bikini Class B Winner

Appendix I
Nutrition Facts and Serving Size

The top half of the Nutrition Facts label gives you serving information. The serving information shows the serving size and the number of servings contained in the product. This is key because the information that you learn from the rest of the label depends on the serving size. There are two parts to the actual package size; this is not the same as the serving size and can be very misleading. If a package of cookies contains six cookies and a serving size is equal to two cookies, then the entire package contains three servings, not one.

```
              Chicken Noodle Soup
        Nutrition Facts
   Serving Size 1/2 cup (120 ml) condensed soup
   Servings Per Container about 2.5

   Amount Per Serving

   Calories   60        Calories from Fat  15
                                 % Daily Value*
   Total Fat   1.5g                        2%
     Saturated Fat  0.5g                   3%
     Trans Fat  0g
   Cholesterol   15mg
   Sodium   890gm                          37%
   Total Carbohydrate   8g                 3%
     Dietary Fiber   1g                    4%
     Sugars   1g
   Protein   3g

   Vitamin A       4%    Calcium        0%
   Vitamin C       0%    Iron           2%
   *Percent Daily Values are based on a 2,000 calorie diet.
   Your Daily Values may be higher or lower depending on
   your calorie needs.

                  Calories    2000      2500
   Total Fat       Less than   65g       80g
     Sat Fat       Less than   20g       25g
   Cholesterol     Less than  300mg     300mg
   Sodium          Less than  2,400m    2400mg
   Total Carbohydrate         300g      375g
     Dietary Fiber            25g       30g
```

On the chicken noodle soup example here, it is important to note that a serving is one-half cup of the condensed soup directly from the can and not one-half cup of the soup *after* water has been added. Always look at the Nutrition Facts label to see if the serving size should be measured or counted *before* the product is prepared or *after* preparation.

Appendix II
Glossary and Basic Body Poses

Fruit: a usually sweet food (such as a blueberry, orange, apple, or tomato) that grows on a tree or bush. (*Merriam-Webster ELL*; WebMD)

Gluten: a substance in wheat and flour that holds dough together. Gluten is the protein found in wheat, rye, and barley. It is common in most grain-based products, such as cereals, breads, and pasta. Gluten intolerance is characterized by abdominal pain, gas, bloating, and/or diarrhea. Higher-level gluten intolerance is considered celiac disease, when the presence of gluten triggers the body's immune system. Eating foods or using products containing gluten may cause an individual's immune system to respond by damaging the villi, the tiny, fingerlike projections in the small intestine that absorb the nutrients from food. (*Merriam Webster ELL*; WebMD

Basic Body Poses for Reference

Round Shape Examples
- Start by lying on your back. Extend your legs and your arms upward. Slowly stretch and see if you can touch your hands to your toes.
- Start by standing and facing your parent or guardian. Extend your hands upward to touch their hands. Slowly round your back while your parent/guardian does the same to form a circle.

Cube (Box) Example
- Get down on your hands and knees, and keep your back flat to form a cube (box).

Visit your local library or go online to find additional shapes/body poses you can make with your body for fun.

Appendix III
Additional Resources from
http://www.choosemyplate.gov/index.html

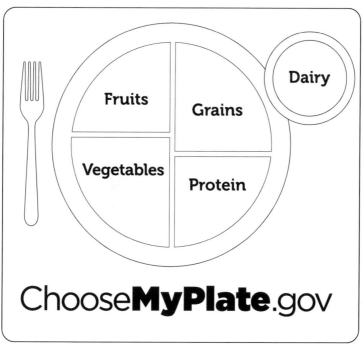

MyPyramid Worksheet

Name: _____

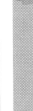

MyPyramid FOR KIDS

Check how you did yesterday and set a goal to aim for tomorrow

Write In Your Choices From Yesterday	Food and Activity	Tip	Goal (Based On a 1800 Calorie Pattern)	List Each Food Choice In Its Food Group*	Estimate Your Total
Breakfast:	**Grains**	Make at least half your grains whole grains.	**6 ounce equivalents** (1 ounce equivalent is about 1 slice bread, 1 cup dry cereal, or ½ cup cooked rice, pasta, or cereal)		____ ounce equivalents
Lunch:	**Vegetables**	Color your plate with all kinds of great tasting veggies.	**2½ cups** (Choose from dark green, orange, starchy, dry beans and peas, or other veggies).		____ cups
Snack:	**Fruits**	Make most choices fruit, not juice.	**1½ cups**		____ cups
Dinner:	**Milk**	Choose fat-free or lowfat most often.	**3 cups** (1 cup yogurt or 1½ ounces cheese = 1 cup milk)		____ cups
	Meat and Beans	Choose lean meat and chicken or turkey. Vary your choices--more fish, beans, peas, nuts, and seeds.	**5 ounce equivalents** (1 ounce equivalent is 1 ounce meat, chicken or turkey, or fish, 1 egg, 1 T. peanut butter, ½ ounce nuts, or ¼ cup dry beans)		____ ounce equivalents
Physical activity:	**Physical Activity**	Build more physical activity into your daily routine at home and school.	At least **60 minutes** of moderate to vigorous activity a day or most days.		____ minutes

*Some foods don't fit into any group. These "extras" may be mainly fat or sugar—limit your intake of these.

How did you do yesterday? ☐ Great ☐ So-So ☐ Not So Great

My food goal for tomorrow is: _____

My activity goal for tomorrow is: _____

10 tips

MyPyramid
Nutrition Education Series

cut back on sweet treats

10 tips to cut back on added sugars

Cut back on buying foods and beverages with added sugars. If you don't buy them, your kids won't get them very often. Eating too many sweet treats can contribute to tooth decay and overweight. So, it is important for kids, and adults, to limit eating sugary foods and drinks.

1 serve small portions
It's not necessary to get rid of all sweets and desserts. Instead, teach your child that a small amount of sweets or a treat can go a long ways. Use smaller bowls, plates, and utensils for your child to eat with. Children can practice serving from small bowls as you help them.

2 skip the soda
Soda is high in calories and contains a lot of sugar. Skip the store's soda or sweetened beverage aisle completely. Remind your child that you've already picked out a juice together. Make fresh fruit smoothies together by blending fresh or frozen fruit with fat-free or low-fat milk and yogurt or 100% juice.

3 use the check-out lane that does not display candy
Most grocery stores will have a candy-free check-out lane to help moms out. Waiting in a store line makes it easy for children to ask for the candy or gum that is right in front of their faces to tempt them.

4 choose not to offer sweets as rewards
By offering food as a reward for good behavior, children learn to think that some foods are better than other foods. Reward your child with kind words and comforting hugs or non-food items, like stickers, to make them feel special.

5 offer fruit for dessert
Serve baked apples, pears, or enjoy a fruit salad. Or, serve yummy frozen juice bars (100% juice) as a healthy option instead of high-fat desserts.

6 make food fun
Sugary foods that are marketed to kids are advertised as "fun foods." Try making nutritious foods fun by preparing them with your child's help and being creative together. Make a smiley face with sliced bananas for eyes, raisins for a nose, and an orange slice for a mouth. Or, cut fruit into fun and easy shapes with cookie cutters.

7 encourage children to invent new snacks
Make your own trail mixes from dry cereal, dried fruit, and nuts or seeds. Provide them with a table full of fresh and nutritious foods, and allow children to pick and choose what they want in their "new" innovative snack.

8 name a food your child helps make
Serve "Dawn's Salad" or "Peter's Sweet Potatoes" for dinner. The food will be nutritious and your child will be proud of the meal he or she helped create. They will also be more willing to try new things if they get involved in meal planning.

9 play with food
Let your child make towers out of whole-grain crackers or make funny faces on plates with pieces of fruit.

10 if meals are not eaten, kids do not need "extras"
Candy or cookies are not replacements for foods not eaten at meal times.

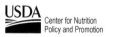

Center for Nutrition
Policy and Promotion

Go to MyPyramid.gov for more information.

Nutrition TipSheet No. 8
November 2009
USDA is an equal opportunity provider and employer.

41

Cucumber Yogurt Dip

Serving Size: 1/6 of recipe

Yield: 6 servings

Ingredients:

2 large cucumbers

2 cups plain yogurt, low-fat

½ cup sour cream, non-fat

1 tablespoon lemon juice

1 tablespoon fresh dill

1 garlic clove, chopped

1 cup cherry tomatoes

1 cup broccoli florets

1 cup baby carrots

Food Group Amounts:

Color	Food Group	Amount
	Grains	--
	Vegetables	1¼ c
	Fruits	--
	Dairy	¼ c
	Protein	0

Nutrient Totals

Per Serving:

Calories	100
Total Fat	1.5 g
Saturated Fat	1 g
Sodium	120 mg
Protein	6 g

Preparation:

1. Peel, seed, and grate one cucumber. Slice other cucumber and set aside.
2. Mix grated cucumber, yogurt, sour cream, lemon juice, dill, and garlic in a serving bowl. Chill for 1 hour.
3. Arrange tomatoes, cucumbers, broccoli, and carrots on a colorful platter.
4. Serve with dip.

Source: SNAP-Ed Connection

Lemon Velvet Supreme

Serving Size: 1/6 of recipe

Yield: 6 servings

Ingredients:

2 cups vanilla yogurt, fat-free

3 tablespoons instant, lemon pudding mix

8 squares graham crackers, crushed

1 can (4 ounces) mandarin orange slices, drained (or your favorite fruit)

Preparation:

1. Combine vanilla yogurt and pudding mix; gently stir together.

2. Layer bottom of serving dish with crushed graham crackers.

3. Pour pudding mixture over cracker crumbs.

4. Top with mandarin orange slices or your favorite fruit.

Source: SNAP-Ed Connection

Food Group Amounts:

Color	Food Group	Amount
	Grains	½ oz
	Vegetables	--
	Fruits	0
	Dairy	¼ c
	Protein	--

Nutrient Totals

Per Serving:

Calories	150
Total Fat	1 g
Saturated Fat	0 g
Sodium	21 mg
Protein	5 g

Corn Chowder

Serving Size: 1 cup
Yield: 4 servings

Food Group Amounts:

Color	Food Group	Amount
	Grains	--
	Vegetables	¾ c
	Fruits	--
	Dairy	½ c
	Protein	--

Nutrient Totals

Per Serving:

Calories	186
Total Fat	5 g
Saturated Fat	1 g
Sodium	205 mg
Protein	7 g

Ingredients:

1 tablespoon vegetable oil

2 tablespoons finely diced celery

2 tablespoons onion, finely diced

2 tablespoons finely diced green pepper

1 package (10 ounces) frozen whole kernel corn

1 cup raw diced potatoes, peeled,

1 cup water

¼ teaspoon salt

Black pepper to taste

¼ teaspoon paprika

2 cups milk, non-fat, divided

2 tablespoons flour

2 tablespoons chopped fresh parsley

Preparation:

1. In medium saucepan, heat oil over medium high heat.
2. Add celery, onion, and green pepper; sauté for 2 minutes.
3. Add corn, potatoes, water, salt, pepper, and paprika. Bring to a boil; reduce heat to medium; and cook, covered, about 10 minutes or until potatoes are tender.
4. Pour ½ cup milk into a jar with a tight-fitting lid. Add flour and shake vigorously.
5. Add gradually to cooked vegetables; stir well.
6. Add remaining milk.
7. Cook, stirring constantly, until mixture comes to a boil and thickens.
8. Serve garnished with chopped fresh parsley.

Source: "A Healthier You." U.S. Department of Health and Human Services.

Zesty Tomato Soup

Serving Size: 1 cup

Yield: 4 servings

Ingredients:

1 can (14.5 ounces) no-salt added diced tomatoes

1 cup roasted red peppers, drained

1 cup evaporated milk, fat-free

1 teaspoon garlic powder

¼ teaspoon ground black pepper

2 tablespoons fresh basil, rinsed and chopped (or 2 teaspoons dried)

Preparation:

1. Combine tomatoes and red peppers in a blender or food processor. Puree until smooth.

2. Put tomato mixture in a medium sauce pan and bring to a boil over medium heat.

3. Add evaporated milk, garlic powder, and pepper. Return to a boil, reduce heat to low, and gently simmer for 5 minutes.

4. Add basil and serve.

Source: SNAP-Ed Connection

Food Group Amounts:

Color	Food Group	Amount
	Grains	--
	Vegetables	¾ c
	Fruits	--
	Dairy	½ c
	Protein	--

Nutrient Totals

Per Serving:

Calories	94
Total Fat	0 g
Saturated Fat	0 g
Sodium	231 mg
Protein	5 g

Outtasight Salad

Serving Size: 1 cup
Yield: 4 servings

Ingredients:

2 cups salad greens of your choice

1 cup chopped vegetables (tomatoes, cucumbers, carrots, green beans)

1 cup juice-packed pineapple chunks, drained, or fresh orange segments

¼ cup Dressing (see below)

2 tablespoons raisins or dried cranberries

2 tablespoons chopped nuts, any kind

Preparation:

1. Put mixed salad greens on a large platter or in a salad bowl.
2. In a large bowl, mix chopped vegetables and pineapple or orange segments.
3. Add dressing and stir.
4. Spoon mixture over salad greens.
5. Top with raisins and nuts.

Dressing:

¼ cup yogurt, nonfat, plain or fruit-flavored

1 tablespoon orange juice

1½ teaspoons white vinegar

Preparation:

1. In a small bowl, mix all ingredients. Refrigerate until ready to serve.

Source: SNAP-Ed Connection

Food Group Amounts:

Color	Food Group	Amount
	Grains	--
	Vegetables	½ c
	Fruits	¼ c
	Dairy	0
	Protein	½ oz

Nutrient Totals

Per Serving:

Calories	100
Total Fat	2.5 g
Saturated Fat	0 g
Sodium	30 mg
Protein	2 g

Roasted Root Vegetables

Serving Size: ¼ cup

Yield: 4 servings

Ingredients:

2 medium-sized sweet potatoes, cut into large chunks

2 medium-sized root vegetables (white potatoes, rutabagas, turnips, parsnips, beets), cut into large chunks

2 carrots, chopped

1 medium onion, chopped

¼ cup vegetable oil

3 tablespoons Parmesan cheese

Season with your favorite spices

Preparation:

1. Preheat oven to 350 degrees F.

2. In a medium bowl, add all chopped vegetables, and pour oil over top.

3. Add Parmesan cheese and seasonings; mix well.

4. Spread vegetable mixture evenly on a baking sheet.

5. Bake for 1 hour or until tender.

Source: SNAP-Ed Connection

Food Group Amounts:

Color	Food Group	Amount
	Grains	--
	Vegetables	1¼ c
	Fruits	--
	Dairy	--
	Protein	--

Nutrient Totals

Per Serving:

Calories	250
Total Fat	15 g
Saturated Fat	2 g
Sodium	150 mg
Protein	5 g

Rise and Shine Breakfast Cobbler

Serving Size: ¾ cup

Yield: 4 servings

Ingredients:

1 cup juice-packed canned sliced peaches, drained

1 cup juice-packed canned sliced pear halves, drained

6 pitted prunes, cut in half (or other dried fruit)

¼ teaspoon vanilla extract

1 orange, zested and juiced

1 cup granola, low-fat

Preparation:

1. In a large microwave-safe bowl, mix peaches, pears, prunes, vanilla extract, orange zest, ¼ cup orange juice; stir.

2. Top with granola.

4. Microwave on high for 5 minutes. Let stand for 2 minutes.

5. Spoon into 4 bowls and serve warm.

Source: SNAP-Ed Connection

Food Group Amounts:		
Color	Food Group	Amount
	Grains	½ oz
	Vegetables	--
	Fruits	1 c
	Dairy	--
	Protein	--

Nutrient Totals

Per Serving:

Calories	280
Total Fat	1 g
Saturated Fat	0 g
Sodium	60 mg
Protein	3 g

Frozen Fruit Cups

Serving Size: 1/18 of recipe
Yield: 18 servings

Ingredients:

3 bananas, mashed

24 ounces yogurt, non-fat strawberry flavored (or plain)

10 ounces strawberries, frozen, thawed, undrained

1 can (8 ounces) crushed pineapple, undrained

Preparation:

1. Line muffin tin(s) cups with paper baking cups (18 total).
2. In a large mixing bowl, add mashed bananas, yogurt, strawberries, and pineapple.
3. Spoon into muffin tin and freeze at least 3 hours or until firm.
5. Remove frozen cups and store in a plastic bag in the freezer.
6. Before serving, remove paper cups.

Source: SNAP-Ed Connection

Food Group Amounts:

Color	Food Group	Amount
	Grains	--
	Vegetables	--
	Fruits	¼ c
	Dairy	¼ c
	Protein	--

Nutrient Totals

Per Serving:

Calories	50
Total Fat	0 g
Saturated Fat	0 g
Sodium	25 mg
Protein	2 g

Fire and Ice Watermelon Salad

Serving Size: 1½ cup

Yield: 4 servings

Ingredients:

6 cups watermelon, rind removed, cut into large chunks

2 green onions, thinly sliced

⅓ cup thinly sliced red onion

⅓ cup torn mint leaves

1 tablespoon red pepper flakes

⅔ cup white vinegar

3 tablespoons vegetable oil

1 tablespoon chili powder

Food Group Amounts:		
Color	Food Group	Amount
	Grains	--
	Vegetables	¼ c
	Fruits	1½ c
	Dairy	--
	Protein	--

Nutrient Totals

Per Serving:

Calories	132
Total Fat	7 g
Saturated Fat	1
Sodium	12 g
Protein	1 g

Preparation:

1. In a large bowl, combine watermelon, onions, mint, and red pepper flakes.

2. In a small bowl, mix vinegar, oil, and chili powder.

3. Drizzle vinegar mixture over watermelon mixture and serve.

Bulgar Chickpea Salad

Yield: 6 servings

Ingredients:

1¼ cups water

1 cup coarse bulgur

1 teaspoon dried parsley

1 teaspoon minced onion

1 teaspoon soy sauce

½ cup chopped green onions

½ cup raisins

½ cup chopped carrots

¾ cup canned chickpeas (garbanzo beans), drained and rinsed

Food Group Amounts:		
Color	Food Group	Amount
	Grains	1½ oz
	Vegetables	¼ c
	Fruits	¼ c
	Dairy	--
	Protein	½ oz

Nutrient Totals

Per Serving:

Calories	200
Total Fat	5 g
Saturated Fat	0.5 g
Sodium	330 mg
Protein	5 g

Dressing:

2 tablespoons oil

2 tablespoons lemon juice

1 tablespoon soy sauce

1 garlic clove, minced

Black pepper to taste

Preparation:

1. In a medium saucepan, bring water to boil. Stir in bulgur, parsley, minced onion, and soy sauce. Reduce heat to low and cover. Simmer 15-20 minutes (until all water is absorbed and bulgur is not too crunchy). Do not overcook.

2. Remove from heat and allow to cool; fluff with fork.

3. Combine dressing ingredients; stir well.

4. Put bulgur mixture in a large bowl. Pour dressing over bulgur mixture and mix well.

5. Stir in green onions, raisins, carrots, and chickpeas. Cover and chill for several hours.

Source: SNAP-Ed Connection

Berry Bread Pudding

Serving Size: 1 cup
Yield: 2 servings

Ingredients:

1½ cups unsweetened, frozen berries, thawed, undrained (or fresh)

   (blueberries, sliced strawberries, or raspberries)

½ teaspoon sugar (optional)

½ teaspoon vanilla extract or almond extract (optional)

4 or 5 slices whole wheat bread, crusts removed

Vanilla yogurt (optional)

Preparation:

1. In a small bowl, combine the thawed berries, sugar and/or vanilla extract.
2. Spoon ¼ cup of the berry mixture to cover the bottom of a 2 cup deep dish.
3. Cover the berry mixture with a layer of bread.
4. Spoon ⅓ of remaining berry mixture on top of the bread.
5. Cover with another layer of bread.
6. Repeat steps 4 and 5 twice ending with a layer of bread.
7. Cover the dish with plastic wrap and place a plate or bowl on top of the berry dish that fits just inside of it. Place a heavy object on top to press down on the fruit and bread layers.
8. Refrigerate overnight. (Check the dish to be sure juice does not run over the top. You may need to replace the heavy object with a lighter one to prevent spills.)
9. Serve with a dollop of vanilla yogurt.

Note: In summer fresh berries can be used.

Food Group Amounts:

Color	Food Group	Amount
	Grains	2 oz
	Vegetables	--
	Fruits	¾ c
	Dairy	--
	Protein	--

Nutrient Totals

Per Serving:

Calories	180
Total Fat	2.5 g
Saturated Fat	0.5 g
Sodium	300 mg
Protein	6 g

Source: SNAP-Ed Connection

Carribbean Casserole

Serving Size: 1 cup
Yield: 10 servings

Ingredients:

1 medium onion, chopped

½ green pepper, diced

1 tablespoon canola oil

1 can (14.5 ounces) stewed tomatoes

1 teaspoon oregano leaves

½ teaspoon garlic powder

1½ cups instant brown rice, uncooked

1 can (16 ounces) black beans, undrained (or beans of your choice)

Food Group Amounts:		
Color	Food Group	Amount
	Grains	1 oz
	Vegetables	¼ c
	Fruits	--
	Dairy	--
	Protein	½ oz

Nutrient Totals

Per Serving:

Calories	100
Total Fat	2 g
Saturated Fat	0 g
Sodium	280 mg
Protein	4 g

Preparation:

1. In a large pan, heat oil over medium heat.

2. Add onion and green pepper in canola oil, in a large pan, and cook until tender. Do not brown.

3. Add tomatoes, beans (include liquid from both), oregano, and garlic powder.

4. Bring to a boil. Stir in rice and cover.

5. Reduce heat to low and cook for 5 minutes.

6. Remove from heat and let stand for 5 minutes before serving.

Source: SNAP-Ed Connection

20-minute Chicken Creole

Serving Size: 1 cup

Yield: 8 servings

Ingredients:

1 tablespoon vegetable oil

2 whole chicken breasts, skinless, boneless, cut into ½-inch strips

1 can (14.5 ounce) diced tomatoes with juice

1 cup chili sauce, low sodium

1 large green pepper, chopped

2 celery stalks, chopped

1 small onion, chopped

2 garlic cloves, minced

1 teaspoon dried basil

1 teaspoon dried parsley

¼ teaspoon cayenne pepper

¼ teaspoon salt

Food Group Amounts:		
Color	Food Group	Amount
	Grains	--
	Vegetables	½ c
	Fruits	--
	Dairy	--
	Protein	1½ oz

Nutrient Totals

Per Serving:

Calories	130
Total Fat	3 g
Saturated Fat	0 g
Sodium	260 mg
Protein	9 g

Preparation:

1. In a large pan, heat oil over medium-high heat.
2. Add chicken and cook 5 minutes, stirring occasionally.
3. Reduce heat to medium and add remaining ingredients.
4. Bring to a boil then reduce heat to low. Simmer, covered for 15 minutes.
5. Serve over hot, cooked rice or whole-wheat pasta.

Source: SNAP-Ed Connection

Lentil Chili

Serving Size: 1 cup
Yield: 6 servings

Ingredients:

½ pound ground beef (Or extra lean beef to reduce fat)

1½ cups chopped onion

1 clove garlic, crushed

2 cups cooked, drained lentils

1 can (29 ounce) tomatoes, diced or crushed

1 tablespoon chili powder

½ teaspoon ground cumin (optional)

Preparation:

1. In a large saucepan, brown beef over medium-high heat, breaking it into bite-sized pieces. Drain fat.
2. Reduce to medium heat. Add onion and garlic. Cook on medium heat, until softened.
3. Add lentils, tomatoes, chili powder, and cumin. Cook on low heat for about 1 hour until flavors are blended.
4. Serve with your favorite chili toppings.

Source: SNAP-Ed Connection

Food Group Amounts:

Color	Food Group	Amount
	Grains	--
	Vegetables	¾ c
	Fruits	--
	Dairy	--
	Protein	2 oz

Nutrient Totals

Per Serving:

Calories	210
Total Fat	4.5 g
Saturated Fat	1.5 g
Sodium	470 mg
Protein	16 g

Salmon Patties

Serving Size: 1/9 of recipe
Yield: 9 servings

Ingredients:

1 can (15½ ounces) salmon, drained

1 cup whole-grain, crushed cereal or crackers

2 large eggs, lightly beaten

½ cup 1% milk

1/8 teaspoon black pepper

1 tablespoon vegetable oil

Preparation:

1. Use a fork or clean fingers to flake salmon until very fine.
2. Crumble cereal or crackers into crumbs.
3. Add cereal or cracker crumbs, eggs, milk, and pepper to salmon.
4. Mix thoroughly.
5. Shape into 9 patties.
6. In a skillet, heat oil over medium heat.
7. Carefully brown both the sides until patty is thoroughly cooked.

Source: SNAP-Ed Connection

Food Group Amounts:

Color	Food Group	Amount
	Grains	½ oz
	Vegetables	--
	Fruits	--
	Dairy	0
	Protein	2 oz

Nutrient Totals

Per Serving:

Calories	110
Total Fat	4.5 g
Saturated Fat	1 g
Sodium	270 mg
Protein	12 g